The Sweet Read
8990 Main Street
Woodstock, GA 30188
678-562-4100
www.thesweetread.com

Praise for *"Secrets of a Successful Loser"*

"What a wealth of information in such a short read! This is the perfect book for managing weight wisely. The writing style is light and whimsical, but packed with sound advice!"
Courtney Bradley, RN, MSN, MNS

"So many diet books are complicated and this is short and sweet. It has good, common sense ideas which are easy to follow. Basically, I think it's a winner!!"
Linda Zeien, MD

"A refreshing and common sense approach to a national epidemic."
R. Mac Chapman, MD

"This book is like a well-built compact car. It drives well, is easy to operate, does not have any flaws, and will get you where you want to go without complications. Dr. Gettys and Dr. Reynolds understand the science of healthy weight loss and have developed a simple and practical plan that anyone can follow."
Rudy Scarfalloto D.C., author of *Nutrition for Massage Therapists, What Should I Eat* and other works.

"I love the book! It allows me to make dieting personal and fit in with my lifestyle. The recipes are good. Also, as I lost weight before, I kept buying clothes as I lost. I never thought of the consignment shop idea. I am very encouraged about starting back on a diet. Thank you for sharing these ideas!"
Pam Sellers, LPN

"Who knows your emotional struggles and feelings about weight loss better than someone who has been there too? And who can help you succeed with your wellness and weight goals better than two passionate women doctors? This is not your typical one size fits all weight loss book. Dr. Katherine Gettys and Dr. Susan Reynolds understand the body from a physician's training — and the struggle with weight and self esteem. This is a fun, self empowering, easy to read weight loss book. You will want to share it with all your friends!"

Stephen C Monahan, life coach and author of *Awakening the Mysterious Feminine*

"Secrets of a Successful Loser was such an easy read and provided great advice and reason for the one and only healthy method for losing weight, which is feeding your body the nutrients it truly needs while also exercising or moving your body in a manner that promotes wellness and the maintenance of a healthy body weight."

Belinthia Poole, RD, LD

"Great book! It shows that weight loss can be successful and healthy—and can be done by anyone."

Cindy Smith, LPN

"This book is highly informative and much needed. It is an honest realistic guide to practical weight loss and maintenance."

Sarah T. Chapman, MA, LPC, LCAS

"Great resource! A simple and practical application for weight loss."

Emmanuel Quaye, M.D., Internal Medicine and Functional Medicine

Secrets of a Successful Loser

The Problems

People Have with Weight Loss...

and *How We've Solved Them*

Katherine Gettys MD and Susan D. Reynolds MD
Illustrations by Katherine Gettys MD

www.secretsofasuccessfulloser.com

Katherine Gettys MD accepts a limited number of speaking engagements each year at conferences, associations, seminars and webinars. Please direct your request to the author by email at gettyskl@gmail.com.

ATTENTION CORPORATIONS, UNIVERSITIES, COLLEGES, AND PROFESSIONAL ORGANIZATIONS: Quantity discounts are available on bulk purchases of this book for educational, gift purposes, or as premiums for increasing magazine subscriptions or renewals. Special books or book excerpts can also be created to fit specific needs. For information, please contact Yawn's Publishing company.

Published by: Yawn's Publishing
210 East Main Street
Canton, GA 30114
www.yawnspublishing.com

This publication contains the opinions and ideas of its authors. It is intended to provide helpful and informative material on the subjects addressed in the publication. It is sold with the understanding that the authors and the publisher are not engaged in rendering medical, health, or any other kind of personal professional services in the book. The reader should consult his or her medical, health, or other competent professional before adopting any of the suggestions in this book or drawing inferences from it.

The authors and publisher specifically disclaim all responsibility for any liability, loss or risk, personal or otherwise, which is incurred as a consequence, directly or indirectly, of the use and application of any of the contents of this book.
Printed in the United States of America

First Printing 2012

ISBN: 978-1-936815-61-6
Library of Congress Control Number: 2012949139

Dedication

This book is dedicated to the women and men who are fighting the battle of the bulge every day.

"Most people are shooting themselves in the foot with a loaded fork."

Katherine Gettys MD

Contents

Introduction

You have tried to lose weight and you know it can be really hard. Maybe you have tried and failed several times. Maybe you have lost the weight then regained all the pounds you lost. Are you are heavier now than when you started dieting? Does this describe you?

It's not your fault.

That's right; it's not your fault. Your body is designed to help you *survive.* Your ancestors made it through the lean times by storing extra calories as fat and living off this fat when food was scarce. Your body is *programmed* to be a fat-storing machine.

This survival mechanism worked great when food was in short supply. But now, in the days of high fat, high sugar, high calorie super-sized meals, what helped your ancestors hurts you. Your body is not meant to be living in this over-abundant food environment.

Our ancestors had it much easier than we do. They didn't have to spend energy and attention to maintain a healthy weight. Physical activity was a part of life and healthy food was their only choice. Sugar was not plentiful and fast food didn't exist so there was no temptation to resist. Their choices were made for them.

Every day you are bombarded by literally thousands of marketing messages and hundreds of unhealthy food choices. Temptation is everywhere and willpower just isn't enough anymore.

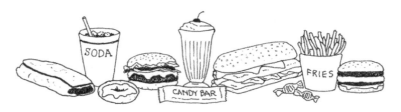

Staying healthy in an unhealthy world means developing a strategy for success. The problems are real but fortunately so are the solutions.

On the following pages are the solutions we developed for our own weight loss problems. Our simple strategies were created by busy doctors and work for busy people like you.

Winning the weight loss battle isn't just about losing weight. It's about being healthy, looking great and feeling energetic. It's about developing habits so the lost pounds don't find you again.

Why bother to lose weight? You've failed so many times before.

Because... Being overweight puts you at risk for type 2 diabetes, hypertension, cardiovascular disease and premature death. In addition, obesity can cause fatty liver (which can lead to cirrhosis), obstructive sleep apnea, gallbladder disease, gastroesophageal reflux disease, certain types of cancer (prostate cancer, uterine cancer, colon cancer and breast cancer), reproductive system disorders, osteoarthritis, gout, deep vein thrombosis, pulmonary embolism, psychological problems, and low self-esteem. If you have high cholesterol or a family history of heart disease and you are a smoker, your chances of getting these diseases are even higher.

Diabetes

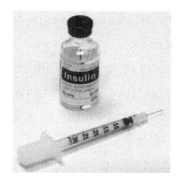

Type 2 diabetes in the United States has reached epidemic proportions. According to the National Institute of Health, 25.8 million Americans of all ages have diabetes. That's 8.3 percent of the U.S. population. Of these, 18.8 million have been diagnosed and 7.0 million are yet unaware of this metabolic time bomb.

Look at these sobering 2010 statistics from The National Institute of Diabetes and Digestive and Kidney Diseases (NIDDK) and National Institutes of Health (NIH):

- Among U.S. residents ages 65 years and older, 10.9 million, or 26.9 percent, had diabetes.

3

- Approximately 215,000 people younger than 20 years had type 1 or type 2 diabetes in the United States.
- About 1.9 million people ages 20 years or older were newly diagnosed with diabetes in the United States.
- Between 2005 and 2008, 35 percent of U.S. adults ages 20 years or older tested positive for prediabetes. Of adults ages 65 years or older, a full half tested positive. Applying this percentage to the entire U.S. population in 2010 yields an estimated 79 million American adults 20 years or older suffering from prediabetes.
- Diabetes is the leading cause of kidney failure, non-accident related leg and foot amputations, and new cases of blindness among adults in the United States.
- Diabetes is a major cause of heart disease and stroke.
- Diabetes is the seventh leading cause of death in the United States.

Overall, the risk for death among diabetics is 200% higher than people without diabetes.

Health experts say, if nothing changes, 1/3 of the children born in the year 2000 will develop diabetes. Currently about

¼ of teenagers with type 2 diabetes already have signs of neuropathy which puts them at very high risk of leg amputation.

Type 1 diabetes, formerly known as *juvenile onset diabetes mellitus*, generally occurs at a younger age than type 2 diabetes and is thought possibly to be caused by an autoimmune reaction following an acute illness. However, **Type 2 diabetes**, previously known as *adult onset diabetes mellitus*, is being caused increasingly by obesity. This is reaching epidemic proportions and is now affecting children as well as adults.

Fortunately, losing even a small amount of weight will lower blood sugar allowing many diabetics to stop taking oral diabetes medication or insulin. If you do have diabetes, monitor your blood sugar closely and work with your doctor to adjust your medications and improve dietary habits.

High Blood Pressure

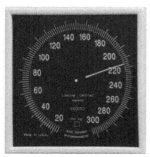

Being overweight causes blood pressure to rise. High blood pressure or hypertension has been called "the silent killer." Many people who have it don't know it until something catastrophic (such as a stroke or a heart attack) happens.

5

When you are overweight, even if you are not a diabetic, your cells become less sensitive to insulin so you need more insulin to do the same job. Your pancreas produces more insulin. This extra insulin tells your kidneys to hold on to sodium and water. With more sodium and water in your circulatory system, your blood pressure goes up. It's a simple equation:

Excess weight + excess insulin = more sodium retention

+ high blood pressure

Approximately 80% of diabetics have high blood pressure. High blood pressure increases your chances of having a stroke, heart attack, kidney disease and damage to other organs.

The good news is that weight loss will naturally lower your blood pressure. (So will regular exercise.) If you currently take blood pressure medication, you may notice that you require a lower dose as you lose weight. It may be possible for some people to get off of blood pressure medication entirely. Be sure to work with your doctor to have your medicine adjusted properly.

Now that you know the dangers of excess weight, let's explore the solutions!

Chapter 1

Before You Start

"There are no shortcuts to any place worth going."
Beverly Sills

Your ultimate goal is a healthy weight but first you have to determine *what is a healthy weight for you.* People have different body types. It has been said that people are built like spaghetti, linguini or fettuccini. Some of us will always be stocky like a fettuccini noodle. Others have a slender build like spaghetti.

Whatever your build, the goal is to decrease your body fat to a healthy level.

Body Mass Index

First, let's assess where you are now. The easiest way is to use a scale, a measuring tape and a Body Mass Index (BMI) chart. Doctors use your BMI to determine if you are in an underweight, normal, overweight or obese category. Your BMI is calculated from your weight and height and provides an estimation of your body fat. It is the recommended way of expressing weight relative to height for adults.

> BMI is defined as the weight in kilograms divided by the square of the height in meters.

BMI calculation has its limitations as a tool. It is not always accurate in certain populations such as children, the elderly, certain ethnic groups such as Asians, muscular athletes and people who have lost a lot of muscle mass. If you have a lot of muscle, your BMI measurement may overestimate your body fat. Conversely if you have lost and regained weight many times, you probably lost muscle so your BMI may underestimate the amount of fat.

Write your height and weight below:

My height:_____

My weight:_____

Now, use the BMI chart on the next page to determine your Body Mass Index.

My BMI:_____

The National Institute of Health has the following classifications:

BMI less than 18.5 = underweight

BMI 18.5 to 24.9 = normal

BMI 25 to 29.9 = overweight

BMI 30 and above = obesity

As your weight rises above normal, your health declines. If you have a BMI over 40, you have an extremely high risk for disease.

	Normal			Overweight				Obese											Extreme Obesity			
BMI	23	24	25	26	27	28	29	30	31	32	33	34	35	36	37	38	39	40	41	42	43
Height (inches)								Body weight (pounds)														
58	110	115	119	124	129	134	138	143	148	153	158	162	167	172	177	181	186	191	196	201	205
59	114	119	124	128	133	138	143	148	153	158	163	168	173	178	183	188	193	198	203	208	212
60	118	123	128	133	138	143	148	153	158	163	168	174	179	184	189	194	199	204	209	215	220
61	122	127	132	137	143	148	153	158	164	169	174	180	185	190	195	201	206	211	217	222	227
62	126	131	136	142	147	153	158	164	169	175	180	186	191	196	202	207	213	218	224	229	235
63	130	135	141	146	152	157	163	169	175	180	186	191	197	203	208	214	220	225	231	237	242
64	134	140	145	151	157	163	169	174	180	186	192	197	204	209	215	221	227	232	238	244	250
65	138	144	150	156	162	168	174	180	186	192	198	204	210	216	222	228	234	240	246	252	258
66	142	148	155	161	167	173	179	186	192	198	204	210	216	223	229	235	241	247	253	260	266
67	146	153	159	166	172	178	185	191	198	204	211	217	223	230	236	242	249	255	261	268	274
68	151	158	164	171	177	184	190	197	203	210	216	223	230	236	243	249	256	262	269	276	282
69	155	162	169	176	182	189	196	203	209	216	223	230	236	243	250	257	263	270	278	284	291
70	160	167	174	181	188	195	202	209	216	222	229	236	243	250	257	264	271	278	285	292	299
71	165	172	179	186	193	200	208	215	222	229	236	243	250	257	265	272	279	286	293	301	308
72	169	177	184	191	199	206	213	221	228	235	242	250	258	265	272	279	287	294	302	309	316
73	174	182	189	197	204	212	219	227	235	242	250	257	265	272	280	288	295	302	310	318	325
74	179	186	194	202	210	218	225	233	241	249	256	264	272	280	287	295	303	311	319	326	334
75	184	192	200	208	216	224	232	240	248	256	264	272	279	287	295	303	311	319	327	335	343
76	189	197	205	213	221	230	238	246	254	263	271	279	287	295	304	312	320	328	336	344	353

BMI chart (data from the National Institute of Health)

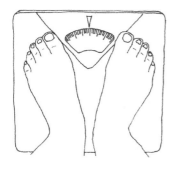 Your scale is your friend, not your enemy. People who weigh themselves on a regular basis have an easier time losing weight and keeping it off. Your scale can help keep you accountable. Watching the numbers on your scale go down shows how much you have accomplished!

Waist circumference

If you carry most of your weight around your waist, you have a greater chance of developing heart disease than someone who carries weight primarily in the hips and thighs. Women with a waist size of **greater than 35 inches** and men with a waist size of **greater than 40 inches** are more likely to develop heart disease and type II diabetes than people with smaller waist sizes.

My waist circumference is _____ inches.

How much weight do you need to lose?

Even losing only a small amount of weight will help you lower the risk of developing some of these weight related diseases. Depending on your current weight, a loss of as little as 10 pounds can markedly improve your health.

You can determine your ideal weight for your height from the BMI chart or from checking the ideal weight for height chart below:

Height	Weight in Pounds
4'10"	91-119
4'11"	94-124
5'0"	97-128
5'1"	101-132
5'2"	104-137
5'3"	107-141
5'4"	111-146
5'5"	114-150
5'6"	118-155
5'7"	121-160
5'8"	125-164
5'9"	129-169
5'10"	132-174
5'11"	136-179
6'0"	140-184
6'1"	144-189
6'2"	148-195
6'3"	152-200
6'4"	156-205
6'5"	160-211
6'6"	164-216

Source: Evidence Report of Clinical Guidelines on the Identification, Evaluation, and Treatment of Overweight and Obesity in Adults, 1998. NIH/National Heart, Lung, and Blood Institute (NHLBI).

My ideal weight is:_____

I need to lose _____ pounds.

How many calories do you need to eat?

Your calorie needs are determined by your Basal Metabolic Rate (BMR). Your BMR includes the calories you spend on basic body functions like breathing and circulation as well as the calories you use for daily activities. If you are very active and spend a lot of your time on your feet, you need more calories than someone who spends most of his or her time sitting.

Your BMR is determined by multiplying your current body weight times 10.

For example, an average 150 pound woman needs 1500 calories a day to maintain her weight. (150 x 10 = 1500)

My BMR: My weight_____ x 10 =_____calories

If our 150 pound woman is an athlete such as a long distance runner, she will need many more calories to maintain the same weight.

To determine how many calories you need to eat in a day to lose weight, a good estimation is to multiply your *ideal* weight by 10. If you weigh 180 pounds and your ideal weight is 140 pounds, you should be eating 140 x 10 or 1400 calories.

My ideal caloric intake:

My ideal weight_____ x 10 =_____calories

To increase the calories your body burns every day, you can also increase your daily activity level. However, it's a lot easier to not eat 500 calories than it is to burn 500 calories from exercise.

Activities which will burn 500 calories:

- Riding on a stationary bike at a moderate pace for 1 hour 15 minutes
- Using a stair climbing machine for 55 minutes
- Low impact aerobics for 1 hour 40 minutes
- Water aerobics for 2 hours
- Walking at a moderate pace for 2 ½ hours

Exercise is a great thing to do for so many reasons but losing weight isn't one of them. *At least 80%* of your body composition is determined by what you eat. If you are tired and overweight and just cannot face the idea of exercise, the good news is changing your diet alone can get you where you want to go. As you lose weight, your energy will increase and then you can start exercising.

Exercise has a very important role in maintaining your weight loss and building back some of the muscle you lost. When you lose weight on a typical diet, two-thirds of the weight you lose is fat and one-third is lean body mass, essentially muscle. Unfortunately, if you gain the weight back, 80% of the weight you regain is fat and only 20% is muscle.

Yo-yo dieting, losing then regaining weight several times, has a terrible effect on your body composition.

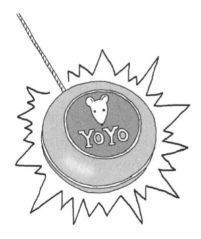

Your metabolism becomes slower since you have less muscle so it becomes harder and harder to lose weight. Exercise, particularly resistance exercise like weight training, can change this. You can add back all the muscle you have lost and speed up your metabolism so it's easier to keep the weight off.

A note about diet pills

Grocery store shelves are filled with pills that promise quick and easy weight loss. Most over the counter products claim to be appetite suppressants or thermogenic aids. (A thermogenic aid claims to speed up metabolism to help you burn more calories.) It sounds tempting but none of these have ever been proven to help in sustaining long term weight loss and all of them have side effects. Do you remember ephedrine? Ephedrine was widely used as an over the counter appetite suppressant and weight loss aid for decades until the FDA banned its use in weight loss drugs in 2004. It has some of the same effects as amphetamines and was associated with heart problems and several deaths.

Prescription drugs aren't much better. Most FDA approved weight loss drugs (appetite suppressants) are meant to be used for a very brief period of time – only weeks to months. People rapidly develop tolerance to these drugs which lose their effectiveness as a result. When folks stop taking these drugs, their appetites return and weight gain quickly follows. Unfortunately, many people regain more weight than they lost.

Some of these drugs or drug combinations have been proven over time to be dangerous. Phen/Fen was a combination of two appetite suppressant drugs Phentermine and Fenfluramine. It was heavily marketed in the late 1990's until physicians began seeing cases of heart valve damage and pulmonary hypertension primarily in women who had taken the drugs. Fenfluramine was found to be the culprit and the drug combination was taken off the market, unfortunately not before many people developed significant health problems.

Orlistat (also called Xenical or Alli) is currently the only weight loss drug approved for long term use. It has no effect on appetite. Xenical is prescribed for people who have a significant amount of weight to lose and studies have shown it to be safe for up to 2 years. Alli (half the strength of Xenical) is available over the counter. Both medications block the absorption of about 30% of dietary fat.

Dieters who take Orlistat, follow a healthy diet, and exercise may lose more weight than those who only use diet and exercise alone. However Orlistat does have some side effects including malabsorption of fat-soluble vitamins D, A, K and E. Dieters who use Orlistat need to take a daily multivitamin or a whole food supplement such as Juice Plus+ to replace the vitamins that may be lost in the stool. It is also advised that they follow a low fat diet to minimize side effects such as loose or oily stools. However, these side effects indicate that the drug is working as it prevents absorption of fats. The drug itself passes straight through the GI tract with only traces (almost none) being absorbed into the body.

The FDA has recently approved new diet drugs. They have significant side effects and contraindications. There are no studies demonstrating long term safety or effectiveness.

Remember that ALL drugs have side effects. Familiarize yourself with any drug that you take.

Laxatives and diuretics (water pills) are not a safe way to lose weight. They can cause dehydration and electrolyte imbalances. Besides that, you are not losing fat with these drugs. You are only losing valuable body fluids and minerals.

Your goal is to lose fat and keep it off *for good* while preserving muscle mass. Losing weight will have a tremendous impact on your health but only if you don't gain the weight back. We are doctors and will share our weight loss strategies and secrets for keeping it off. You'll learn a lifelong plan that doesn't involve deprivation or spending all your spare time in a gym.

Soon YOU can celebrate becoming a *successful loser!*

Chapter 2

Master Your Motivation

"Ability is what you're capable of doing. Motivation determines what you do. Attitude determines how well you do it."
Raymond Chandler

"Believe in yourself! Have faith in your abilities! Without a humble but reasonable confidence in your own powers you cannot be successful or happy."
Norman Vincent Peale

"Desire is the key to motivation, but it's determination and commitment to an unrelenting pursuit of your goal - a commitment to excellence - that will enable you to attain

the success you seek."
Mario Andretti

Does this sound like you? "I need to lose weight but I'm just can't get started."

Everybody struggles with getting started but people who set and accomplish goals have found a way to get and stay motivated.

You know why you *need* to lose weight. It's important to prevent diabetes or avoid complications of diabetes. Weight loss will help reduce your risk of cancer, reduce your risk of heart disease and improve symptoms of arthritis. These are all very important reasons but often they are not enough.

A more important reason is why do you *want* to lose weight?

Successful dieters are no different from you. Their secret is that they have identified their "why". When your "why" is strong enough, you will have all the motivation you need to make the necessary changes.

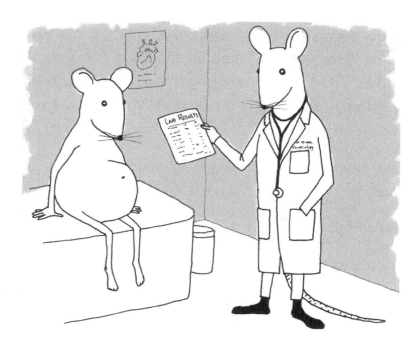

Let's get started!

What is your "why?"

Many people find their why in their important relationships. Who is important to you?

_____

Do you have children or a spouse who depend on you?

Do you have parents who are concerned about you?

Sometimes it's easier to do something for someone else than it is to do it for yourself. Think of the times you went to work when you weren't feeling well. Or when you went without sleep to take care of a sick child. You did what you had to do for them.

You are important to the people in your life. Think of someone who would really miss you if you were gone.

Who is depending on you?

It's much easier to do anything if you have support or a partner. Who can help you achieve your weight loss goals?_____

_____

When can you talk to them about helping you achieve your goals? (Write down a date and a time)

_____

What do you want to accomplish in your life?

_____

_____

How do you want people to remember you after you are gone?

_____

_____

What do you want to do that you are not doing now because of your weight?

_____

_____

_____

How would it feel to do this thing? (Write the answer to this question in detail)

_____

_____

_____

How will your life be different when you have lost the weight?

_____

_____

_____

Describe how you will feel when you accomplish your weight loss goal?

_____

_____

_____

_____

How will you feel if you do not accomplish this goal?

_____

_____

_____

Think back on an accomplishment that is important to you.

I accomplished

_____

_____

_____

What were the obstacles you overcame to achieve your goal?

_____

_____

_____

What were the strengths you used to get through these obstacles?

_____

_____

_____

How can you use these strengths to help you achieve your weight loss goal?

_____

_____

_____

What are 3 obstacles in the way of your successful weight loss?

1._____

2._____

3._____

List at least 3 strategies to overcome each obstacle.

1._____

_____

_____

2._____

_____

_____

3._____

_____

_____

Visualize how you will look and feel when you are at your ideal weight. Spend some time and create a clear mental picture.

What clothes will you wear?

_____

_____

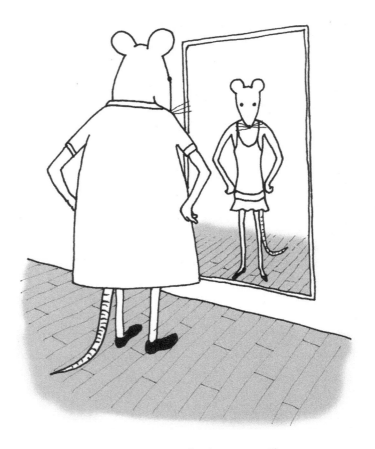

I'm going to look so good!

What will you do?

_____

_____

How will you feel?

_____

_____

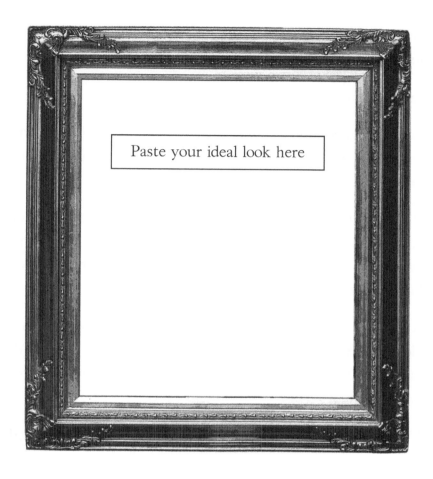

Paste your ideal look here

Wow, you look magnificent!

Keep that picture in your mind. Your subconscious mind will help you achieve your goals.

> When your why is big enough, the how will take care of itself.

Set up your reward system

Looking good and feeling great is the reward you will experience when you have lost weight. But what are your rewards along the way?

It can be hard to get motivated because all you can think of are the things you can't do now and the rewards you aren't getting in the present while the payoff for changing your habits is still in the future.

It is important to reward yourself for your accomplishments along the way. We need rewards to keep us motivated. All habits, good or bad, are based on getting a reward after we have taken an action.

If there is no reward, it will be too hard to take sustained action.

About Habits

Scientists say you can never get rid of a bad habit. That sounds like really bad news. But is it? The good news is while you can't get rid of a bad habit, you can change it into a good habit.

A habit loop begins with a *cue* or *trigger* that leads to taking an *action* which is followed by a *reward*. This is how humans (and dogs and cats and horses) operate.

You will always have cues or triggers and you will always need rewards. However you can change your actions in response to triggers and you can develop different rewards.

Nancy's Story

Let's use Nancy as an example. She started going by a fast food restaurant on the way home from work and ordering a hamburger and fries with a large soda. Her cue was leaving work and passing the restaurant on the way home. Her action was ordering the hamburger and fries and her reward was eating the unhealthy food.

Over a period of 10 years, she gained 75 pounds.

Eventually her health began to suffer and she knew she needed to change her unhealthy habits.

She looked at some of the habits which had led to her weight gain. The first habit she decided to change was her fast food habit.

On weekdays when she left work, she took a different route home so she avoided the fast food restaurant. She started meeting a friend at a park near her house and they walked 2 miles every day after work. When she came home, she made a delicious berry shake.

Nancy's Protein Shake

8 oz. unsweetened vanilla almond milk

4 frozen strawberries

¼ cup frozen blueberries

1 scoop vanilla Juice Plus+ Complete powder

3 ice cubes

Put all ingredients in blender and blend.

Nancy avoided temptation by not driving by the fast food restaurant. She found a walking partner who kept her accountable. And she had a delicious meal after her walk.

Nancy's cue or trigger for her bad habit was leaving work and driving by the fast food restaurant. She still had the cue of leaving work but she avoided temptation by changing her route home.

Her previous action was buying and eating fast food in her car.

Her new action was meeting a friend and walking in the park. She substituted a healthy action for an unhealthy one. After a short period of time, as she lost weight and got more fit, she began to consider the walk itself as part of her reward.

After the walk, she drank a smoothie which substituted for the previous reward, the fast food and soda.

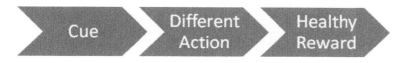

Think of some of your habits. What is your cue to act and what is the reward you get for taking the action?

_____

_____

_____

Which unhealthy habit can you change first?

_____

Which unhealthy habit can you change next?

_____

After you start changing your habits, you will begin to lose weight without struggling.

What is your reward going to be when you have lost 5 pounds?

_____

When you have lost 10 pounds?

_____

When you have lost 20 pounds?

_____

Chapter 3

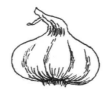

Success Strategies

Have you ever said...

"I'm really confused about all the diet advice out there."

"I don't know how to cook."

Join the crowd! You hear a lot of conflicting information about food and nutrition. The thing is, the human body hasn't changed in thousands of years. Your body has certain needs that only real food, not processed food, can provide.

Keep it simple.

Eating well doesn't have to be complicated or expensive. In fact healthy food is often easier and cheaper.

Here are some of our favorite, simple solutions to help you eat better and live better.

1. Food Labels

Know what you're eating. This means reading food labels. If you need a degree in organic chemistry to understand what you are eating, maybe you should skip it!
Read the entire food label. Pay special attention to the portion size at the top of the label. Maybe the food only has 70 calories but the serving size is unrealistically small.

Notice not only the calories from fat but the type of fat. Some fats are worse than others. Trans fat is not safe in any amount. A labeling loophole allows food manufactures to call a food "trans fat free" if there is less than 0.5g of trans fat per serving. Beware! If you read the fine print at the bottom of the label and-see any "partially hydrogenated oil", such as soybean or cottonseed, it is a trans fat.

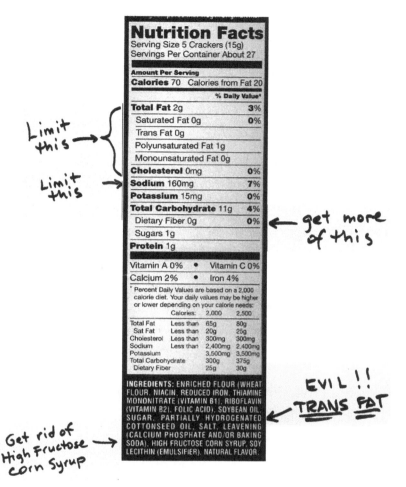

Always read the fine print!

Also look for high fructose corn syrup. This ever-present sugar is a big contributor to Americans' expanding waistlines.

2. Real Food

Eat real food. Graze on greens, not high calorie snacks. Fill up on a rainbow of healthy vegetables and fruits. When you eat real food, not processed food, you know what you are getting.

When you eat real food you are also getting all of the nutrients your body needs. Vegetables and fruits contain tens of thousands of phytonutrients, healthy chemicals which act synergistically to help your health.

Chronic inflammation is at the root of most of the diseases seen in industrialized nations. Stress, a poor diet and being overweight increase inflammation.

Good news! Phytonutrients, nutrients from vegetables and fruits, reduce inflammation. People who eat the highest number of servings of vegetables and fruits have lower rates of heart disease, cancer, stroke and diabetes. They also live longer.

Foods that have been processed then fortified or enriched with 12 vitamins can't compare with the nutrient density of broccoli or cabbage or blueberries. Processed foods also lack water and fiber so they don't fill you up prompting over eating.

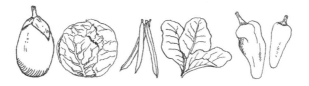

Shop around the edges of the grocery store, in the produce and meat and dairy sections. Avoid the center aisles filled with processed foods and empty calories.

3. Protein

Eat enough protein. Researchers have found that people have a large appetite for protein. When the ratio of protein to fat and carbohydrates is too low, they tend to overeat.

In one study, volunteers consumed more calories when they were on a 10% protein diet than when they were on a diet containing 15% to 25% protein. Most of the extra calories came from snacks rather than from healthy, balanced meals.

As we age, our bodies are less efficient in absorbing and using dietary protein so older people need *more* protein than younger people. Unfortunately often we get less protein than we need.

Your body needs protein to repair and maintain all of your organs and tissues, including your liver, kidneys, digestive tract and heart. Your muscle has the largest amount of protein and functions as a protein "bank." Over time, if you consume less protein than your body needs to maintain healthy organs, your body will start withdrawing amino acids (the building blocks of protein). This breaking down of your muscle tissue leads to something called "sarcopenia," or muscle wasting. This leads to weakness, frailty and eventually loss of mobility.

Aim for 30 grams of protein per meal in at least 2 and hopefully 3 meals a day. A great meal contains a serving of lean protein and 2 to 3 servings of different vegetables and fruit. The good news is this kind of meal is very filling and satisfying.

What does 30 grams of protein look like?
- a 6 oz can of tuna or salmon
-1 cup of lowfat cottage cheese
-1 ½ cups plain Greek yogurt
-1 cup liquid egg substitute
-5 oz baked flounder or pollock
-5 cups of regular oatmeal
-5 cups of Raisin Bran cereal
-1 ½ cups raw almonds

-1 block tofu

-2 cups cooked black or kidney beans

-4 oz broiled sirloin steak

-4 oz pork loin

-5 oz roasted chicken breast

-3 chicken drumsticks

-4 oz roasted turkey

-5 cups cooked spinach

(from USDA Bulletin, Nutritive Value of Foods)

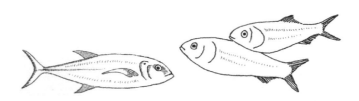

4. Fluid Calories

Don't drink your calories. Sodas and sugary drinks are some of the biggest causes of weight gain and one of the easiest things to change. Your body doesn't react to calories in thin liquids the way it reacts to solid food or thick liquids such as soup or smoothies. What's different? Your stomach doesn't give you the signal that it's full so it's easy to consume hundreds of extra calories.

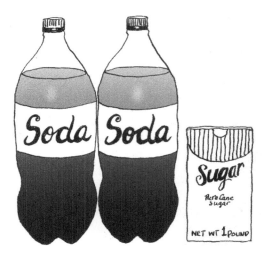

Two 2 liter sodas contain a FULL POUND of sugar!

Fruit juice has a lot of natural fruit sugar but doesn't have any of the fruit fiber which slows down the absorption of sugar into the bloodstream. You will get a sugar spike followed by a sugar crash which will make you feel tired and hungry. Eating whole fruit is a much better idea. Eating an apple is much more filling than merely drinking apple juice.

Watch out for energy drinks as well as sodas and juices. Many energy drinks are full of sugar and caffeine. You will get an initial energy burst but it won't be sustained. The caffeine can cause dehydration which will make you feel worse than before you drank the energy drink.

Diet drinks eliminate sugar and calories, but better choices for beverages would be water or unsweetened green, black or oolong tea which contain powerful antioxidants called catechins. Catechins work like vitamin C and vitamin E in food to block damage to your cells caused by oxidative stress.

Some studies have shown a reduced risk of several cancers including skin, colon and breast cancer among regular tea drinkers. Drinking tea can also help reduce your risk of heart disease by stopping the oxidation of LDL cholesterol. Oxidized LDL damages blood vessel walls and leads to atherosclerotic heart disease and high blood pressure.

Diet sodas have no calories but they also have no nutritional value. Unsweetened fruit juice or skim milk have some nutritional value but it is still best to avoid drinking calories if you are trying to lose weight.

5. Develop the water habit.

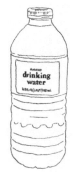

Carry a bottle filled with water and sip on it all day. Staying hydrated can keep you from feeling tired.

Drink water when you are feeling hungry. Often we mistake thirst for hunger.

The amount of water you need to drink depends on your environment and your activity level.

To monitor your water needs, examine your urine. It should be pale yellow. If it is dark yellow, you may not be drinking enough water.

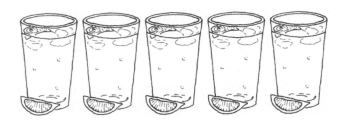

6. Eat breakfast.

This is critical. Your body has fasted overnight and really needs a morning protein boost. *Give it what it needs.* Research proves that people who eat breakfast consume fewer calories throughout the day.

And, make sure you eat the *right kind* of breakfast.

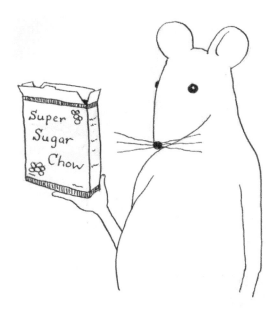

No wonder I'm hungry again in an hour.

Many Breakfast cereals contain as much sugar as a candy bar but they don't contain very much protein.

If you don't get enough protein for breakfast, you will feel hungry quickly and will tend to eat unhealthy snacks to tide you over to lunch.

7. Snack, but snack sensibly.

You can't feel hungry all the time and expect to maintain that forever. When you are hungry, eat.

Keep healthy snacks with you *all the time*. It's too easy to grab the first thing you see in the vending machine if you get too hungry.

Smart snacks:

- Nuts, especially pistachios and walnuts. Both have healthy fats and protein.

A note on pistachios: pistachios have more fiber than most nuts and are packed with high-quality protein. Their heart-healthy unsaturated fats help lower cholesterol which lowers the risk of heart disease and stroke. They also have about half the calories of other nuts. Pistachios in the shell take more time to eat and removing the shells burns calories!
A serving size of sixteen nuts contains only 55 calories.

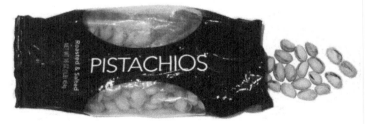

- Sunflower or pumpkin seeds
- Celery, carrots or bell peppers with hummus.
- Hard boiled eggs

- Lettuce wraps with lean uncured deli meat, cheese and a pickle slice
- Cottage cheese or unsweetened Greek yogurt

8. Just say no to sugar.

Sugar by any other name is still sugar and it has a disastrous impact on your body. Sugar is evil. Avoid table sugar, high fructose corn syrup, corn syrup, fructose, agave nectar and honey.

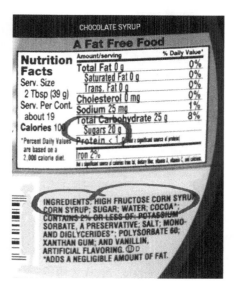

2 tablespoons of chocolate syrup contains enough sugar to increase inflammation in your body for several hours.

Sugar is an addictive food that causes diabetes, promotes cancer and suppresses your immune system. There is no nutritional value in sugar and your body doesn't need it.

150 pounds of sugar

Americans consume
100 to 150 pounds
of sugar a year.

This is way
too much.

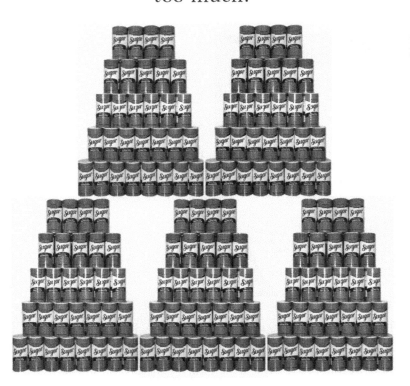

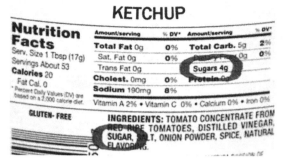

Watch out for hidden sugars. A serving of ketchup contains as much sugar as 1/3 of a bar of Lindt 85% Dark Chocolate. When choosing a candy bar, you expect to be eating sugar; with ketchup, you don't.

9. Eat when it's time, don't eat when it's not.

It's easier to lose weight and maintain that loss when you get most of your calories earlier in the day. Eat breakfast, lunch, dinner and a couple of healthy snacks. Don't eat most of your calories at night for two reasons: 1. you're going to bed and you will be burning the fewest calories. 2. your willpower is less at night and you will be more likely to overeat.

Three eating patterns to avoid:

1. **Binge eating** is the fast consumption of large amounts of food. People who binge report a loss of self-control during the binge and feelings of regret afterward.

2. **Night eating** involves fasting during the early part of the day and eating large amounts of food at night. Up to 50% of the daily food intake may occur after the evening meal. Many people who skip breakfast complain of the urge to eat at night.

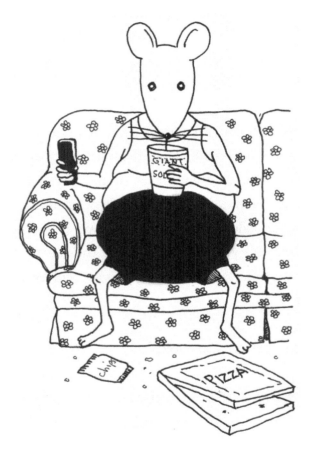

What am I going to eat during the second part of this double feature?

3. **Mindless eating** involves consumption of huge amounts of calories while focusing on something other than the food. For example, many people consume excess calories while sitting in front of the TV. It's too easy to eat more than you need if you are focused on something else, rather than on your food.

When you are eating, make sure it's for the right reason: you are physically hungry, not bored, not dehydrated, not stressed.

Don't eat at your computer or in front of your TV or in bed or any other place where you are *paying attention to something else.*

10. Lose the stress, lose the weight.

Stress causes weight gain and makes it harder to lose weight. Feeling pressured and stressed also undermines your willpower and makes you more likely to give in to emotional eating.

Pay attention to how you feel when you get an urge to eat. Do you feel hunger pangs in your stomach or is your urge coming from your head?

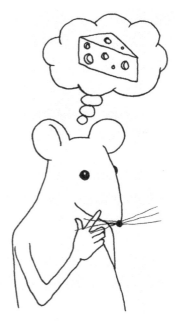

Am I really hungry?

Nadine's strategy

Nadine knows she often eats for emotional reasons. She has found a way to beat this habit by telling herself to wait 30 minutes before eating. "I know I can make it for 30 minutes. I'm not going to starve to death. I'll check in 30 minutes but by then I've usually gotten busy and forgotten about it," says Nadine.

11. Be careful with portions and proportions.

Make at least half of what is on your plate vegetables. Limit fruits and starches such as potatoes and grains until you are close to your weight loss goal.

We suggest you use a small plate. When you use a large plate, it's too tempting to fill the plate with food.

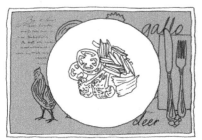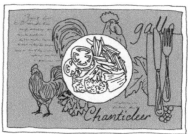

The same amount of food is on both of these plates even though the small plate looks like it contains more food.

When you use a smaller plate, even if you fill your plate, your portion size is automatically limited. You'll eat less by adopting a healthy habit instead of using willpower. Remember you don't have to clean your plate!

12. All calories are not created equal

Some foods are high in sugar and fat and low in nutritional value. They have little fiber or protein and often very little water. These "empty" calories not only don't fill you up but they make you crave more of them.

Some foods, such as sugar, stimulate the pleasure centers in our brains the same way recreational drugs do. Because of this effect, many people say they are "addicted" to certain foods. When they try to stop eating these foods, they get cravings and other withdrawal symptoms.

Foods that contain 200 calories:

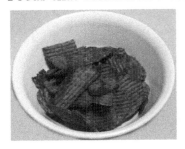

a) Potato chips

1 serving is 1 ¼ oz. (35.4 grams), a small bag or about 25 chips
Calories from fat 110
Total fat 12g
Total carbohydrate 19g
Dietary fiber 1g
Sugars 1g
Protein 2g

A handful of 49 pistachios has about the same number of calories as 13 potato chips.

Or...

b) Wild Alaskan Salmon Salad

1 serving includes 4 oz. canned salmon AND 2 cups of lettuce
Calories from fat 60
Total fat 6g
Total carbohydrate 5g
Dietary fiber 2g
Sugars 0g
Protein 26g

Or...

c) Scrambled Eggs with Spinach, Peppers and Onions

1 serving includes 2 eggs and a half cup each of spinach, peppers and onions
Calories from fat 90
Total fat 10g
Total carbohydrate 8g
Dietary fiber 3g
Sugars 1g
Protein 12g

Which 200 calories is more satisfying?
The salmon salad and scrambled eggs are full meals. They contain healthy fats, a significant amount of protein and

abundant phytonutrients from the vegetables. Vegetables also have fiber and water, both of which fill you up. They will sustain your energy for hours so you won't have a sudden energy crash or cravings.

Potato chips and candy bars aren't meals. Eating them will make you eat more calories because you aren't giving your body what it needs. Your body will send you the signal "Feed me!" even though you just ate because it did not get the nutrition it needed. This is one of the causes of over eating!

13. Plan, Prepare Pack
Plan your menus for the week and do all your shopping at once. Prepare some of your meals on the weekend and freeze them for later. Pack your lunch and your snacks.

Packing your lunch keeps temptation at bay. You know what you are eating and can control your portion size. It also saves time and money.

Controlled snacking will help you keep from getting too hungry and will rev up your metabolism between meals. When you have healthy food available, you are much less likely to give in to temptation.

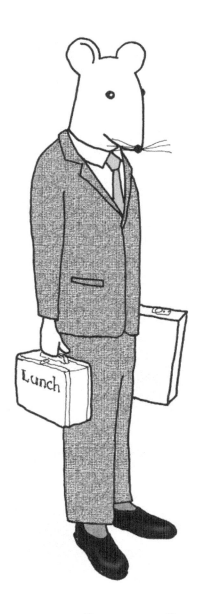

I'm prepared!

"When we talk about planning healthy meals for weight loss, the key point is the planning. You have to take the time to plan ahead so that you are not tempted to pick up the quickest thing at the fast food restaurant or to buy the highly processed foods to prepare at home that take little to no time to put on your table. Your goal should be to eat a variety of foods from all your food groups. Instead of trying to be so complicated in our approach we just need to get back to the basics of cooking a healthy meal at home. Something as simple as a grilled or baked chicken breast, brown rice and a tossed salad with fruit for dessert is a quick and easy meal to put on the table. One of the things that I have found to be the most helpful is to plan your meals for the week and then write your grocery list. This way you only buy what you need and you only prepare what you plan. That helps to eliminate the impulse purchases and puts you a step in the right direction towards a healthier week for you and your family."

Kimberly Alton, RD, LD

Carolina Pines Regional Medical Center,
Hartsville, SC

14. Fiber is your friend.

Fiber fills you up and helps with your digestion.

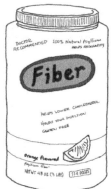

Drink soluble fiber 20 minutes before a meal. This will help your stomach feel full and prevent you from overeating. Soluble fiber like the psyllium in Metamucil® also helps lower cholesterol.

Eat lots of vegetables. In fact the more vegetables you eat, the more easily you will lose weight and keep it off. The fiber and water in vegetables and fruit is more filling than processed food which usually lacks both.

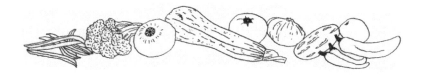

If you eat grains, make sure they are whole grains with fiber rather than heavily processed grains.

Rethinking gluten: Many people have undiagnosed celiac disease or gluten intolerance caused by an autoimmune reaction to gluten, the protein found in wheat, rye and barley. We are eating a lot more gluten, mainly in processed foods, than we did 30 or 40 years ago and sensitivities to gluten are skyrocketing.

Many people find they lose weight immediately and effortlessly when they stop eating gluten. Also many foods containing gluten are processed foods high in sugar and low in nutritional value.

Giving up gluten may be worth a try, particularly if you have been having any digestive problems or recurring skin rashes.

15. Partner with a friend.

Anything is more fun with a friend and you can use the buddy system to keep each other accountable.

Maybe you have a spouse or a friend who needs to lose weight too. Maybe you can start a weight loss group at your job or your church.

You gained weight because of our unhealthy food environment. It's easier to lose the weight in a healthy food environment. What can you do to change your food environment from unhealthy to healthy?

Who can be your partner?

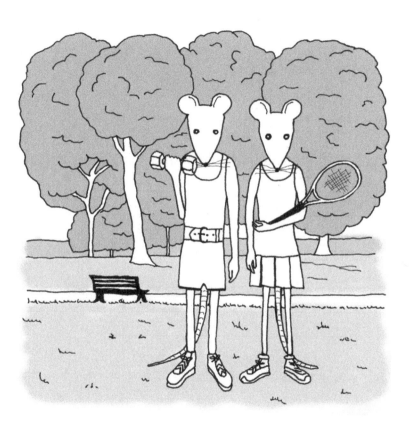

Let's go, partner!

16. Happiness is good for your health.

Happy people are more likely to adopt healthy habits so they live longer.

What makes you happy?

_____

_____

_____

What can you do to add more happy moments to your life?

_____

_____

_____

What is missing in your life now?

_____

_____

_____

How can you get what is missing?

_____

_____

_____

Chapter 4

Time Saving Tips

Do you need a solution to these problems?

"I would like to eat more home cooked meals but I don't have time to do all the shopping and meal preparation."

"I would like to exercise but between my job, my commute and my family, I don't have the time."

Most of us have too little time and too much to do. When we do have the time, we are often too tired to face another chore.

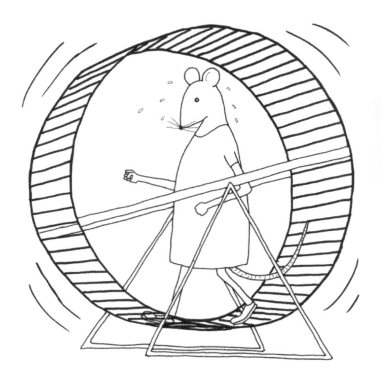

Too much to do. Not enough time.

Fixing great food doesn't have to take a lot of time, especially if you prepare meals in advance. What are some of your favorite healthy meals and snacks? Would it take much more time to make a large batch and freeze some for later?

Often it actually takes less time to create a healthy meal at home than it does to eat out. When you factor in driving time and waiting time, dining out may take longer. When you add in the cost of gas and the food, eating at home is much less expensive. While it is tempting to eat out because someone else is doing the food preparation and clean-up, food preparation does not have to be that time consuming -- with the examples below -- and there are always paper plates.

The next time you go out to eat, make a note of the time it takes and how much it costs. The answer may surprise you.

Mexican dinner at a local restaurant:

22 minutes driving time, to and from the restaurant
25 minutes from arrival at restaurant to receiving food
15 minutes to eat
Total time: 1 hour, 2 minutes
Cost: $1.50 gas
$11.50 entrée
$2.50 tip
Total cost: $15.50 *for one person*

Rotisserie chicken dinner at home:

Stop at local grocery store on the way home from work.
15 minutes in grocery store.
2 minutes to put a piece of chicken and salad mix on plate.
15 minutes to eat.
2 minutes to rinse plates and put in dishwasher.
Total time: 34 minutes

Cost: $4.99 rotisserie chicken

$3.49 bag of salad mix with dressing

Total cost: $8.48 *for two people*

Additional time: 10 minutes to take remaining chicken meat off the bones. 10 minutes to make chicken salad out of the leftover chicken. 2 hours to boil chicken bones. 2 minutes to strain chicken broth into container. 30 minutes to make soup using homemade chicken broth. Yield: 4 additional meals.

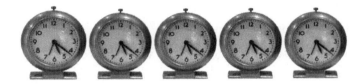

Restaurant and fast food meals are designed to keep customers coming back, not to keep them healthy. They are notoriously high in fat, salt, sugar and calories. In addition, the portion sizes have become much larger in the last decade.

One of the best ways not to overeat is to either split an entrée with a dining partner or to get a takeout container and place at least half of your entree in it before you begin eating.

It is possible to eat a healthy meal in a restaurant but you have to be very careful what you order. Even salads and fish can have enough fattening additions to be unhealthy. Also calorie counts typically underestimate the number of calories in restaurant and fast food.

It pays to eat at home for so many reasons, not just the initial cost of the food. When you make it yourself, you know what's in it.

The NEAT solution

Your grandmother didn't run marathons. She didn't have to. Our generation is the first to have to take time out of the day to do something physical. Before televisions, computers and sedentary jobs, people burned hundreds if not thousands of calories just by going about their daily activities.

Many people think of exercise as a dirty word so let's get rid of it. Let's call it "activity" instead.

Your great-grandparents burned their calories without going to the gym. They did what Dr. James Levine at the Mayo clinic has called NEAT or *Non-Exercise Activity Thermogenesis*. NEAT simply means all the activities you do during the day that burn calories, things like grocery shopping, walking to your car, washing dishes or mowing the lawn.

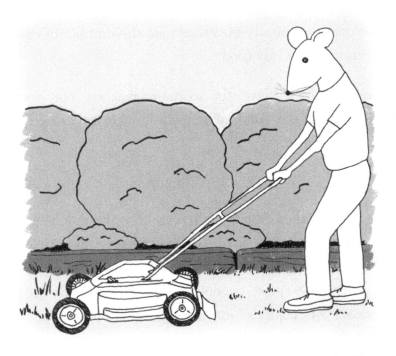

Isn't this more productive than running on a treadmill at the gym?

It's amazing how many calories you can burn without thinking about it by just going about your daily life. For example, a 185 pound person will burn about 200 calories in 30 minutes of raking the lawn, cleaning the gutters or washing the car.

The problem is, most jobs and leisure activities today are sedentary. Our grandparents didn't sit in front of a TV or computer screen all day. They often walked to get where they were going. And they didn't have all the labor saving devices we use for our household chores.

We sit more than any other generation. And *sitting is hazardous to your health!*

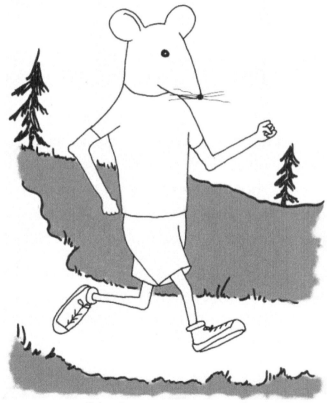

It's time to get moving!

The more standing and moving you do, the more calories you will burn. Computer work burns about 50 calories in a half hour compared to about 90 calories for bartending. A construction worker burns about 200 calories in the same time a truck driver burns about 75.

Walking burns about 4 times as many calories as sitting and merely standing up more often during the workday can burn hundreds of calories a week. (Harvard Medical School, the Harvard Heart Letter, July 2004.)

Small changes in your daily activities can burn hundreds of calories a day, *without going to the gym or exercising!*

Taking the stairs burns more calories than using the elevator. Pacing while talking on the phone burns more calories than sitting. Mowing your lawn with a push mower burns more calories than using a riding lawnmower. Reading burns more calories than watching TV. (Watching TV burns only a few more calories than sleeping.)

What can you do to add more calorie burning activities to your day? Small changes over time make a big difference!

Do you hire someone to mow your lawn? Do it yourself and burn 324 calories an hour.

How about washing your car? This burns 334 calories an hour and costs a lot less than taking it to a car wash.

Heat with a fire? Chopping and splitting wood burns 446 calories an hour.

No wonder our ancestors didn't have to go to the gym!

The NEAT sheet: Engineer your environment to burn more calories during an average day

I sit an average of _____ hours a day.

I walk an average of _____ minutes a day.

I have the following hobbies:

_____

_____

I do the following activities every week: (Vacuuming, laundry, cleaning, and washing the car burn lots of calories.)

_____

_____

_____

What can you change in your office to get more NEAT? List things like rearranging your supplies so you have to stand up to get frequently used items or walking for part of your lunch hour.

10 NEAT strategies at work:

1._____

2._____

3._____

4._____

5._____

6._____

7._____

8._____

9._____

10._____

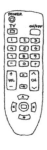 What can you change at home to get more NEAT? List things like Velcroing your remote control to your TV so you have to stand and walk to change the channel.

10 NEAT strategies at home:

1._____

2._____

3._____

4._____

5._____

6._____

7._____

8._____

9._____

10._____

One of the best strategies to increase your activity is to get a pedometer. A pedometer is a great accountability partner. It keeps track of how many steps you took during your day or how many miles you walked. Pedometers are inexpensive and you can get them at department stores as well as sporting goods stores.

Work up to 10,000 steps a day.

When can you start? My start date is:_____

Keep an activity journal and write down your pedometer readings daily. (Your Activity log is in Appendix 3)

Chapter 5

Use Healthy Habits, Not Willpower

"I can resist everything except temptation" Oscar Wilde, *Lady Windermere's Fan*

"Fall seven times, stand up eight."
Japanese proverb

Have you ever said these?

"I keep gaining back all the weight I lost because I don't have any willpower."

"When I see food I love I just can't stop myself from eating it."

Everyone has triggers that undermine willpower. And willpower is not always as strong as we would like it to be.

Willpower is like a muscle; it can get tired. Researchers have found that willpower gets used up during the day. As a result, you have less willpower later in the day. It's no coincidence that many people take in the majority of their calories at night.

Fortunately there are many strategies you can use to help you become a successful loser.

Don't resist temptation; avoid it

There is a reason recovering alcoholics don't spend their spare time in bars. If they did, what are the chances they would start drinking again? It's as unrealistic to expect you to resist the temptation of your favorite fattening foods if they are right in front of you as it is to expect an alcoholic to remain sober while surrounded by alcohol.

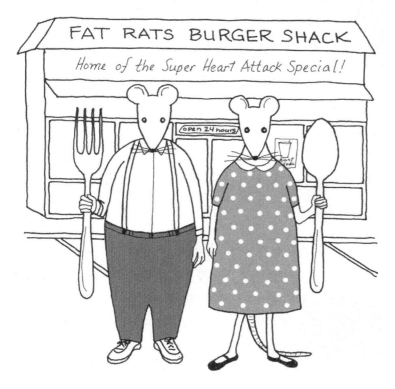

Let's go shovel down some chow!

Our diet is a social phenomenon. We eat what our family and friends eat. We eat what is comfortable, and familiar and available. If the only thing that is available in your environment is junk, then that is what you will eat. Avoid temptation and get rid of addictive food.

Studies show, when it comes to food, "out of sight, out of mind" works. When unhealthy foods are out of sight, we don't crave them the way we do when we see them. Even looking at pictures of fattening, unhealthy foods can cause us to crave them. Keep apples and bananas on the counter and potato chips locked away.

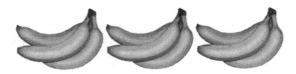

Some foods are trigger foods. These dangerous foods get us started down the slippery slope of binge eating or night eating. Merely having ice cream in the freezer can be enough to derail your diet and negate all the healthy food choices you made during the day.

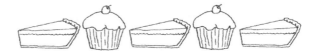

Create a "success kitchen" by purging your refrigerator, freezer and cabinets of your trigger foods. Put your spouse's or kids' snack foods someplace difficult to access. (Actually if these foods aren't healthy, then why are your family members eating them?)

Get Enough Sleep

Recent research shows that sleep deprivation makes people less able to resist the temptation of high calorie foods. When you get less than seven to nine hours of sleep, your hunger hormones get out of whack. You make more ghrelin, the hormone which makes you hungry and less leptin, the hormone which promotes satiety. You will crave sugary foods and have less willpower available to resist the cravings.

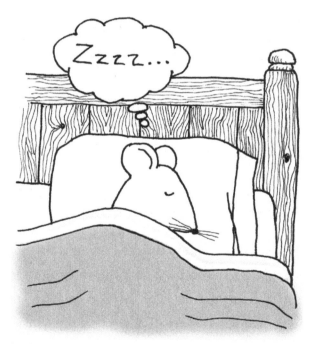

Early to bed, early to rise keeps a mouse healthy!

Rely on Habits, Not Willpower

Do you brush your teeth at night before bed? Is it a huge effort? Brushing your teeth is a healthy habit. It's just something you do without thinking too much about it.

> Success tip: Try brushing your teeth earlier in the evening. Then don't eat anything afterwards.

Create a structure that makes eating healthy food a habit, not an effort of will.

Plan, Prepare, Pack

Plan your meals, prepare your food, pack your snacks. It is much easier to eat a healthy diet if you plan your meals. People who have lost weight and kept it off say this is the key to their success. This way you can control how many calories you are eating at a sitting and you can make sure you have something to eat when you are hungry.

Work with Your Energy, Not Against It

Cook on the weekends and at times when you have the energy. Keep prepared food around so when you are tired, you can grab something healthy. Structure your meals so you don't have to spend a lot of time cooking when you are too tired.

If you don't work with your energy, eventually you will get tired, run out of willpower and indulge in fattening convenience food.

Have Fun

Partner with a friend to be more active. Take ballroom dancing or sign up for an exercise class. If you are having a good time, you will be much more likely to continue moving.

Americans have a fun deficit. If you aren't having enough fun in your life, it will be hard to give up your favorite comfort foods.

What do you do for fun?

_____

What activities did you like when you were a kid?

_____

Why did you like these activities?

_____

What can you do now to experience some of the same joyful feelings?

_____

_____

Weigh Yourself Regularly and Keep Records

When you see the pounds creeping up again, you can cut out some of the foods that are causing you to gain weight. Weigh yourself daily, first thing in the morning, without clothes and before eating. This is your lowest and most accurate weight.

Record your weight on the calendar *every day*. Try to lose 1 to 2 pounds every week until you reach your target weight. When you weigh yourself daily, you can quickly see which foods you need to limit or even eliminate.

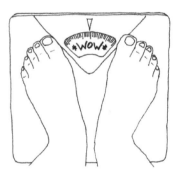

We live in a toxic food environment. Maintaining a healthy weight is a process, not a destination. We may arrive there but it takes attention and vigilance to stay there.

When you have reached your target weight, continue to weigh yourself regularly.

Keep a Food Journal

A food journal acts like an accountability coach. Keeping a record of what you eat keeps eating in check. People who write down what they eat, lose twice as much weight as those who don't.

Awareness is one of the biggest keys to losing weight and keeping it off. Mindless eating is the enemy of your healthy weight. The act of writing down what you are eating makes eating a mindful rather than a mindless act. Your perception and therefore your actions will change.

Eat When You Are Hungry

When you are too hungry, your willpower is lower and you are more likely to eat the first thing at hand, usually an unhealthy convenience food. Twelve step programs use an acronym called HALT. This stands for hungry, angry, lonely or tired. When you feel this way, temptation seems greater than your willpower can handle.

Don't get too hungry. It's hard to resist temptation when you are extremely hungry. Keep healthy snacks like nuts or fat free Greek yogurt or chopped vegetables on hand.

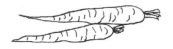

Eat Mindfully

Guard against emotional eating. Why are you really eating? Are you actually hungry or are you just sad, lonely or stressed?

Forgive Yourself

If you fall off your diet, be gentle to yourself. This is natural and it happens to everyone. Just restart the next day. Yes, you do get a do-over.

If you find yourself cheating frequently, try Victoria's strategy.

Victoria's secret

Victoria is a single parent who raised three children by herself. When her youngest child entered his senior year of high school, Victoria decided to lose the 60 extra pounds that had crept up over 15 years of unrelenting stress.

Her success strategy involved creative cheating by designating a "cheat day." During the week, every time she had a food craving, she wrote it in her food journal. On her weekly cheat day, she ate the foods on her list.

Her once a week cheat day kept her motivated the other six days of the week and she has lost a total of 55 pounds in the last 7 months!

Reward Yourself

Give yourself small rewards after achieving small goals. Small goals are attainable and regular rewards help keep you motivated. Researchers have found small rewards given frequently work better than large rewards given infrequently only after achieving large goals.

Nicole's Success Strategy

Nicole has a family and a demanding business. When her youngest son was born, she was in her 40's and 75 pounds overweight. She decided to lose the weight for the sake of her son.

Her hectic schedule left her no "me time." She decided to reward herself every day by taking 30 minutes to go to Starbucks and indulge in a skinny latte.

Nicole says this half hour of uninterrupted time has made it possible for her to stay on her diet and lose 40 pounds.

Choose your rewards wisely. When you first start losing weight, it's tempting to go out and buy new clothes. And you should, but don't spend too much and don't buy too many clothes. They won't fit you for long!

Shoes on the other hand...

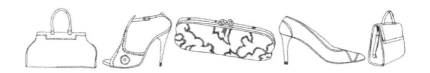

Consignment stores are great places to buy good clothes. And when you have lost another clothing size, you can take the clothes back to where you bought them for someone else to enjoy.

Reward yourself often -- but not with food! Treat yourself with a special gift or sign up for a class you have been wanting to take. Try a weekend getaway with a friend. Pat yourself on the back for a job well done. Celebrate your success.

Chapter 6

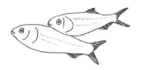

What to eat

"It's difficult to think anything but pleasant thoughts while eating a homegrown tomato."
Lewis Grizzard

"Tell me what you eat, I'll tell you who you are. " Anthelme Brillat-Savarin

"The more you eat, the less flavor; the less you eat, the more flavor."
Chinese Proverb

When you go into a grocery store, you are confronted with an unimaginable array of food choices, most of which are unhealthy. While some choice is good, researchers have found that too many choices makes us unhappy.

Barry Schwartz, the author of *The Paradox of Choice*, described the array of choices he found on a trip to his local grocery store:

85 varieties of crackers
285 varieties of cookies
165 different juice drinks
40 types of toothpaste
360 types of shampoo, conditioner, gel and mousse
275 varieties of cereal
175 varieties of salad dressing

No wonder so many of us are tired and unhappy!

Your ancestors didn't have to spend as much time and energy making choices as you do today. Each choice you make takes time and energy.

When you are tired, under stress or distracted, you tend to buy more and make less healthy choices. This is one of the reasons it's important to shop *at the right time.*

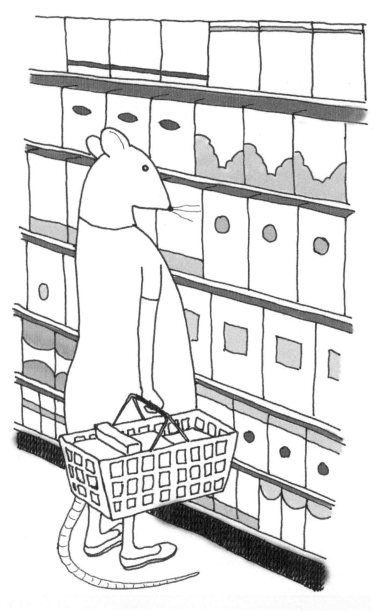

So many choices, all of them of them bad!

Successful shopping tips:
- Always have a list
- Set an alarm on your phone to help you keep your shopping session short
- *Never* shop when you are hungry
- Meditate before you go in the store (people who meditate regularly have more willpower and are less distracted)

Because you live in such a different and more difficult environment than your ancestors, you will not have the luxury of the effortless weight management your grandparents did.

You have to have a strategy to lose weight now and keep it off for a lifetime. One of the success strategies people use is to have a repertoire of simple healthy meals they eat on a regular basis like the recipes in this book.

These meals don't take too much time, thought or energy to make. They are versatile enough that they can be varied with small changes in the basic ingredients. They are good enough to eat not only while you are losing weight but after you have lost it.

Breakfast

Breakfast is the most important meal of the day. Starting the day with a powerful punch of protein sets you up to succeed.

For the first few months, we recommend starting every day with a protein smoothie. This makes it easy to control portions and get enough protein and nutrients.

Protein smoothies also make a quick on-the-go lunch or dinner if you don't have the time or energy to cook.

Protein Smoothie

8 oz. unsweetened vanilla almond milk
1 scoop vanilla Juice Plus+ Complete*
½ scoop vanilla protein powder
¼ cup blueberries**
½ cup crushed ice
Directions:
Put in blender and blend.
(Approximately 250 calories and 30 grams of protein)

*Juice Plus+ Complete is an all-natural plant-based powdered drink mix, not just a protein powder. It contains a blend of plant proteins, 8 grams of fiber and juice powders.

**Variations: Other fruits such as fresh or frozen strawberries, bananas, peaches or frozen fruit blend for smoothies

Cocoa powder with Stevia as a sweetener

Cocoa powder and 1 tbsp almond butter or peppermint extract

Add 1 tbsp ground flaxseeds for a boost of healthy omega 3 fats

Eggs contain healthy fats and protein. They are easy to cook and are amazingly versatile. Omelets and frittatas are as good for dinner as they are for breakfast. Hard boiled eggs make a great snack.

Scrambled eggs with spinach, peppers and onions

2 eggs, beaten

¼ cup diced onion

¼ cup diced bell pepper

½ cup fresh spinach leaves

1 tbsp feta cheese

Dash of garlic powder

Coconut oil

Directions:

Saute onions and bell peppers in coconut oil. Add spinach and garlic powder. When spinach is wilted, stir in eggs and feta cheese. (Under 300 calories)

Hint: Save chopped fresh vegetables from dinner the night before to use in the scramble. Substitute fresh salsa or Pico de gallo for the vegetables

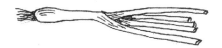

Main meals

Eat *unlimited amounts* of vegetables. Limit fruit consumption until you are closer to your goal weight. Avoid processed and starchy carbohydrates such as potatoes and white flour. Avoid sugar like the plague.

Make sure to eat enough protein or you will have more food cravings and will tend to eat more starchy carbohydrates. Avoid processed meats as they contain preservatives which have been associated with an increased risk of certain types of cancer.

One of the healthiest (and easiest) habits to adopt for a lifetime is to eat a salad every day. Top mixed fresh greens such as baby spring mix, romaine lettuce or spinach with a simple homemade sugar free dressing and diced lean meat or fish. We like to use canned salmon for an omega-3 boost but tuna, shrimp, chicken, pork or beef also work very well.

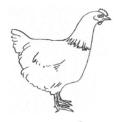 Always keep a source of protein around for a quick meal. Poach several chicken breasts at a time and save extras for lunch the next day. Keeping food like this in your refrigerator will help you stay on track.

Simple Salad Dressing

½ cup distilled red wine vinegar
¼ cup extra virgin olive oil
1 tsp Dijon mustard
½ tsp dill
½ tsp Italian seasoning
1 clove fresh garlic, minced or pressed
Dash of sea salt and fresh ground pepper, optional
Directions:
Add all ingredients to jar. Shake well before using. Keeps several weeks.
(For a more tangy dressing, use white vinegar and cheap yellow mustard instead of red wine vinegar and Dijon mustard. This variation is excellent with chopped pork.)

Salad ingredients:

Mixed salad greens such as spinach, romaine, red leaf or green leaf lettuce
Avocados

Feta cheese
Onions and green onions
Cilantro
Bell peppers
Tomatoes
Radicchio
Arugula
Parsley
Cabbage

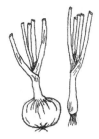

Holiday red and green salad

8 cups mixed romaine lettuce and spinach
1 small head radicchio, chopped
¼ cup cranberries
1/3 cup chopped pecans or walnuts
¼ cup crumbled feta cheese
2 tbsp diced red onion
Directions:
Layer ingredients in a large serving bowl.
Serve with simple salad dressing.
Serves 4 as a side dish, 2 as a main dish salad.

Traditional sandwiches are convenient but eating too much bread can sabotage your diet. A lower calorie alternative is to use lettuce leaves instead of bread.

Lettuce wrap

1-2 lettuce leaves (red leaf, green leaf, romaine)
1 tsp low-calorie mayonnaise
Grilled, broiled or poached chicken, turkey, beef, pork or salmon
Sliced cheese (optional)
Sliced dill pickles (optional)
Directions:
Spread mayonnaise on lettuce leaves. Layer remaining ingredients in the center. Roll up leaves. This is light, crisp and amazingly refreshing. You can add tomato slices, diced cucumbers, olives, green onions, etc.

Seafood is high in protein, rich in healthy omega 3 fats and low in calories. Keep a bag of cooked shrimp in the freezer for quick and easy meals or for a healthy snack.

Shrimp Tacos with Chipotle Coleslaw

Per serving:
1 large lettuce leaf or corn or low carb flour tortilla
5 large boiled shrimp
1 tbsp chopped fresh cilantro
Chipotle coleslaw (recipe below)
Directions:
Place shrimp on tortilla. Add cilantro and coleslaw.

Chipotle coleslaw

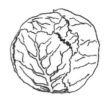

2 cups shredded cabbage

¼ cup finely diced onion

¼ cup low-calorie mayonnaise

1 tsp chipotle Tabasco sauce*

2 tsp fresh lime juice

Directions:

Mix ingredients in a large bowl.

*McIlhenny's Chipotle Tabasco sauce has a mild heat and a smoky flavor.

Beans are one of the best plant-based protein sources. Unlike most other protein sources, they are also very high in fiber and low in fat. Another big advantage is that they are easy to store, whether dried or canned, so you can always keep some around.

Tomato and Black Bean Salad

2 cups diced fresh tomatoes, preferably vine-ripened

1/3 cup diced red onion

¼ cup fresh basil leaves, rinsed and chopped

2 cloves fresh garlic, peeled and chopped or pressed

1 cup cooked or canned black beans, rinsed and drained

¼ cup diced black or Kalamata olives

1 tsp. fresh lemon juice (optional)

2 tbsp. extra virgin olive oil

1 tbsp. red wine vinegar

Fresh ground black pepper

Sea salt to taste

Directions:

Mix all ingredients in large bowl. Top with a little crumbled feta cheese (optional)

One study showed that people consumed fewer calories when their food was prepared as a soup rather than as solid food. Soups are easy to make and freeze well.

Italian Sausage and Bean Soup

4 cups chicken broth

1 pound chicken or turkey Italian sausage, preferably preservative-free

2 cloves garlic, peeled and minced

1 tsp dried basil or 2 tbsp fresh basil

28 oz can of diced tomatoes*

1 can cannellini, great northern, black or kidney beans

Directions:

Remove sausage from casing and brown it in a stockpot. Add garlic and cook 1 minute. Add remaining ingredients and simmer 30 minutes.

*Healthy tips: Grow your own tomatoes or buy fresh tomatoes in season at a farmer's market. Wash and dry the whole tomatoes, then place them in a gallon freezer bag, label and freeze them. They will keep for a year and the peeling protects them from freezer burn. When you defrost them, the peeling will easily slip off.

Wild game and grass-fed beef contain less saturated fat and more healthy omega 3 fat. Recent studies have shown that eating grass-fed lean beef can help people lose weight.

Beef, Turkey or Chicken Chili

1 pound ground or diced lean beef, chicken or turkey

2 onions, chopped

28 oz can of diced tomatoes

2 tbsp chili powder

1 tsp garlic powder or 4 cloves minced garlic

1 can black beans

1 can red kidney beans

Salt and pepper to taste

Directions:

Brown meat in a large stockpot. Add remaining ingredients. Simmer 45 minutes.

At least half of your meal should come from vegetables. Add fruits after you are near your ideal weight as fruit contains a lot of sugar. Avoid dried fruits as they are very high in sugar.

One of the easiest ways to cook vegetables is to roast them.

Roasted Vegetables

Carrots, peeled and sliced
Broccoli and/or cauliflower florets
Brussels sprouts, cut in half
1 small onion, peeled and quartered
Extra virgin olive oil
Sea salt
Fresh ground black pepper or red pepper
Herbes de Provence (or Italian seasoning)

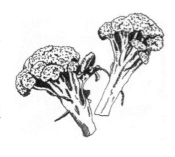

Directions:

Preheat oven to 375º. Drizzle vegetables with olive oil and stir to distribute oil over the surface. Sprinkle with Herbes de Provence. Salt and pepper to taste. Bake 45 minutes, stirring at 15 minute intervals. (You can also roast squash, potatoes or sweet potatoes this way. Peel and cut them into cubes or French fries.)

Kale Chips

Kale leaves washed and torn or cut into 2 inch pieces

Extra virgin olive oil

Sea salt

Directions:

Preheat oven to 375º. Place kale on a cookie sheet and drizzle with olive oil. Toss to coat. Sprinkle with sea salt. Bake 10 to 15 minutes until crispy, checking at 5 minute intervals.

Note: Eat these fresh as they lose their crispness quickly.

How to estimate amounts of food if you can't weigh or measure it:

3 oz. meat is the size of a deck of cards or the palm of an average adult's hand. 3 oz. is half of a small chicken breast or medium pork chop.

1 oz. cheese is the size of your thumb.

1 cup raw leafy greens is the size of your fist.

1/3 cup nuts is a level handful.

½ cup vegetables is 6 asparagus spears, 7 or 8 baby carrots or a medium ear of corn.

Appendix A: Nutrition charts (data from U. S. Department of Agriculture Bulletin Nutritive Value of Foods)

Food	Size	Calories	Protein	Fat	Carbs
Asparagus	1 cup	43	5	1	8
Broccoli	1 cup	25	3	Trace	5
Cabbage	1 cup	18	1	Trace	4
Carrots	1 cup	41	1	Trace	11
Cauliflower	1 cup	25	2	Trace	5
Celery	1 cup	19	1	Trace	4
Cilantro	1 tsp	Trace	Trace	Trace	Trace
Collards	1 cup	49	4	1	9
Corn	1 cup	131	5	1	32
Cucumber	1 cup	14	1	Trace	3
Eggplant	1cup	28	1	Trace	7
Garlic	1 clove	4	Trace	Trace	1
Kale	1 cup	36	2	1	7
Lettuce	1 cup	7	1	Trace	1
Mushrooms	1 cup	18	2	Trace	3
Onions	1 cup	61	2	Trace	14
Bell Pepper	1 cup	40	1	Trace	10
Potato	1 cup	134	3	Trace	31
Soybeans	1 cup	254	22	12	20
Spinach raw	1 cup	7	1	Trace	1
Squash	1 cup	23	1	Trace	5
Tomatoes	1 cup	38	2	1	8
Turnips	1 cup	33	1	Trace	8
Lamb chop	3 oz	219	24	13	0
Chicken Breast	½ breast	142	27	3	0

Food	Size	Calories	Protein	Fat	Carbs
Chicken Thigh	1 thigh	190	13	6	0
Turkey breast	3 oz	133	25	3	0
Turkey dark meat	3 oz	159	24	6	0
Lean Beef	3 oz	213	26	11	0
Pork loin lean	3 oz	172	26	7	0
Ham lean	3 oz	133	21	5	0
Pork sausage	1 patty	100	5	8	Trace
Baked cod	3 oz	89	20	1	0
Salmon baked	3 oz	184	23	9	0
Salmon canned	3 oz	118	17	5	0
Tuna broiled	3 oz	118	25	1	0
Tuna water canned	3 oz	99	22	1	0
Apples	1 apple	81	Trace	Trace	21
Apricots	1 apricot	17	Trace	Trace	4
Avocado	1 oz	50	1	5	2
Banana	1 banana	109	1	1	28
Blueberries	1 cup	81	1	1	20
Cantaloupe	1 cup	56	1	Trace	13

Food	Size	Calories	Protein	Fat	Carbs
Cherries	1 cup	88	2	Trace	22
Cranberries dried	¼ cup	92	Trace	Trace	24
Dates chopped	1 cup	490	4	1	131
Grapefruit	½ fruit	96	1	Trace	9
Grapes	1 cup	114	1	1	28
Grape juice	1 cup	154	1	Trace	38
Lemon	1 lemon	17	Trace	0	5
Lime juice	1 tbsp	3	Trace	Trace	1
Orange	1 orange	62	1	Trace	26
Peaches	1 peach	42	1	Trace	11
Pineapple	1 cup	76	1	1	19
Prunes	5 prunes	100	1	Trace	26
Raisins	1 cup	435	5	1	115
Raspberries frozen	1 cup	258	2	Trace	65
Strawberries raw	1 cup	50	1	Trace	12
Strawberries frozen	1 cup	245	1	Trace	66
Watermelon	1 cup	49	1	1	11
Bagel plain	4" bagel	245	9	1	48
Biscuit	4" biscuit	358	7	16	45

Food	Size	Calories	Protein	Fat	Carbs
Bread wheat	1 slice	65	2	1	12
Bread white	1 slice	67	2	1	12
Corn grits	1 cup	145	3	Trace	31
Oatmeal	1 cup	133	4	1	28
Black beans	1 cup	227	15	1	41
Kidney beans	1 cup	225	15	1	40
Cashews	1 oz	163	4	13	9
Pistachios	47 nuts	161	6	13	8
Almonds	1 oz (24 nuts)	164	6	14	6
Peanut butter	1 tbsp	95	4	8	3
Soy milk	1 cup	81	7	5	4
Soybeans roasted	1 cup	298	29	15	17
Tofu	¼ block	62	7	4	2
Cheddar cheese	1 oz	114	7	9	Trace
Cottage cheese	1 cup	233	28	10	6
Feta	1 oz	49	7	2	1
Mozzarella	1 oz	80	6	6	1
Half and Half	1 tbsp	20	Trace	2	6
Ice cream	½ cup	133	2	7	16

Food	Size	Calories	Protein	Fat	Carbs
Milk whole	1 cup	150	8	8	11
Almond milk*	1 cup	45	1	3	3
Greek yogurt*	1 cup	290	18	23	12
Eggs	1 large	75	6	5	1
Butter	1 tbsp	102	Trace	12	Trace
Olive oil	1 tbsp	119	0	14	0

*Information taken from the package label.

Protein, fat and carbohydrate contents are listed in grams.

www.nal.usda.gov/fnic/foodcomp/Data/HG72/hg72_2002.pdf

Appendix B: Calories burned during daily activities

The following figures are for a 150 pound person:

Activity	Calories burned in 1 hour
Biking (light effort)	409
Dancing (Ballroom, slow)	205
Gardening	324
Golf	240
Light cleaning	240
Cooking	170
Mowing (push mower)	307
Playing with kids	273
Sitting	81
Sleeping	45
Watching TV	72
Strolling	206
Brisk walking	297
Tennis (singles)	545
Vacuuming or mopping	170
Yoga	273
Water Aerobics	477

Sources: Calorie Control Council, American Cancer Society

(http://www.cancer.org/healthy/toolsandcalculators/calculat ors/app/exercise-counts-calculator

http://caloriescount.com/free_getMoving.aspx?AspxAutoDe tectCookieSupport=1

Appendix C: 30 Day Food and activity Log

I will make the 30-day commitment to use this food and activity log to get started on the road to weight loss success *because I'm worth it!*

_____
                    Signature

Start date: _____

Starting weight: _____

Starting waist measurement: _____

Week 1 weight: _____

Week 2 weight: _____

Week 3 weight: _____

Week 4 weight: _____

Week 4 waist measurement: _____

Start date-how I feel:

Week 4-how I feel:

Food and Activity Log

Date	Weight
What I Ate	How I Felt
Breakfast	
Lunch	
Dinner	
Snack	
Activity	Pedometer Reading

Food and Activity Log

Date	Weight
What I Ate	How I felt
Breakfast	
Lunch	
Dinner	
Snack	
Activity	Pedometer Reading

Food and Activity Log

Date	Weight
What I Ate	How I felt
Breakfast	
Lunch	
Dinner	
Snack	
Activity	Pedometer Reading

Food and Activity Log

Date	Weight
What I Ate	How I felt
Breakfast	
Lunch	
Dinner	
Snack	
Activity	Pedometer Reading

Food and Activity Log

Date	Weight
What I Ate	How I felt
Breakfast	
Lunch	
Dinner	
Snack	
Activity	Pedometer Reading

Food and Activity Log

Date	Weight
What I Ate	How I felt
Breakfast	
Lunch	
Dinner	
Snack	
Activity	Pedometer Reading

Food and Activity Log

Date	Weight
What I Ate	How I felt
Breakfast	
Lunch	
Dinner	
Snack	
Activity	Pedometer Reading

Food and Activity Log

Date	Weight
What I Ate	How I felt
Breakfast	
Lunch	
Dinner	
Snack	
Activity	Pedometer Reading

Food and Activity Log

Date	Weight
What I Ate	How I felt
Breakfast	
Lunch	
Dinner	
Snack	
Activity	Pedometer Reading

Food and Activity Log

Date	Weight
What I Ate	How I felt
Breakfast	
Lunch	
Dinner	
Snack	
Activity	Pedometer Reading

Food and Activity Log

Date	Weight
What I Ate	How I felt
Breakfast	
Lunch	
Dinner	
Snack	
Activity	Pedometer Reading

Food and Activity Log

Date	Weight
What I Ate	How I felt
Breakfast	
Lunch	
Dinner	
Snack	
Activity	Pedometer Reading

Food and Activity Log

Date	Weight
What I Ate	How I felt
Breakfast	
Lunch	
Dinner	
Snack	
Activity	Pedometer Reading

Food and Activity Log

Date	Weight
What I Ate	How I felt
Breakfast	
Lunch	
Dinner	
Snack	
Activity	Pedometer Reading

Food and Activity Log

Date	Weight
What I Ate	How I felt
Breakfast	
Lunch	
Dinner	
Snack	
Activity	Pedometer Reading

Food and Activity Log

Date	Weight
What I Ate	How I felt
Breakfast	
Lunch	
Dinner	
Snack	
Activity	Pedometer Reading

Food and Activity Log

Date	Weight
What I Ate	How I felt
Breakfast	
Lunch	
Dinner	
Snack	
Activity	Pedometer Reading

Food and Activity Log

Date	Weight
What I Ate	How I felt
Breakfast	
Lunch	
Dinner	
Snack	
Activity	Pedometer Reading

Food and Activity Log

Date	Weight
What I Ate	How I felt
Breakfast	
Lunch	
Dinner	
Snack	
Activity	Pedometer Reading

Food and Activity Log

Date	Weight
What I Ate	How I felt
Breakfast	
Lunch	
Dinner	
Snack	
Activity	Pedometer Reading

Food and Activity Log

Date	Weight
What I Ate	How I felt
Breakfast	
Lunch	
Dinner	
Snack	
Activity	Pedometer Reading

Food and Activity Log

Date	Weight
What I Ate	How I felt
Breakfast	
Lunch	
Dinner	
Snack	
Activity	Pedometer Reading

Food and Activity Log

Date	Weight
What I Ate	How I felt
Breakfast	
Lunch	
Dinner	
Snack	
Activity	Pedometer Reading

Food and Activity Log

Date	Weight
What I Ate	How I felt
Breakfast	
Lunch	
Dinner	
Snack	
Activity	Pedometer Reading

Food and Activity Log

Date	Weight
What I Ate	How I felt
Breakfast	
Lunch	
Dinner	
Snack	
Activity	Pedometer Reading

Food and Activity Log

Date	Weight
What I Ate	How I felt
Breakfast	
Lunch	
Dinner	
Snack	
Activity	Pedometer Reading

Food and Activity Log

Date	Weight
What I Ate	How I felt
Breakfast	
Lunch	
Dinner	
Snack	
Activity	Pedometer Reading

Food and Activity Log

Date	Weight
What I Ate	How I felt
Breakfast	
Lunch	
Dinner	
Snack	
Activity	Pedometer Reading

Food and Activity Log

Date	Weight
What I Ate	How I felt
Breakfast	
Lunch	
Dinner	
Snack	
Activity	Pedometer Reading

Food and Activity Log

Date	Weight
What I Ate	How I felt
Breakfast	
Lunch	
Dinner	
Snack	
Activity	Pedometer Reading

About the Authors

Katherine Gettys MD and Susan Reynolds MD attended medical school together at the Medical University of South Carolina.

After spending several years performing endocrinology research, Dr. Katherine Gettys did post-graduate work in Pathology at Cedars-Sinai Medical Center in Los Angeles. Over the next 18 years, she saw firsthand the ravages of poor nutrition on the body. As obesity rates skyrocketed and the incidence of obesity-related diseases increased, she switched her focus to wellness and disease prevention. She attended the Institute for Professional Excellence in coaching and is a speaker, author and wellness coach in Canton, Georgia.

After medical school, Dr. Susan D. Reynolds completed 3 years of training in internal medicine (two years at the Medical College of Georgia and one year at the Medical University of South Carolina) and an additional year of training in pathology at MUSC. She has been practicing medicine in the Pee Dee region of South Carolina since 1989. She was voted "Best Family Physician in Darlington County" for 2012. She has witnessed the devastating effects of obesity and wishes to help people overcome this problem.

For more information and resources, visit
www.secretsofasuccessfulloser.com

To order additional copies send check or money order to:

Yawn's Publishing
210 East Main Street
Canton, GA 30114
678-880-1922

___ copies @ _____ each   _____

10% discount on 100 copies   _____

Shipping ($5.00 for up to 6 books) _____

Sales Tax (6%) in Georgia   _____

Total   _____

(allow 2 – 3 weeks for processing)

You may also order with credit card at:

www.yawnspublishing.com

CPSIA information can be obtained at www.ICGtesting.com
Printed in the USA
LVOW022224161112

307750LV00001B/5/P